I0419916

Her Personal Medical Journal

Things Your Doctor Needs to Know

MARY ANN MORROW

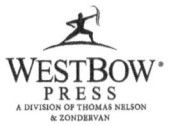

WESTBOW®
PRESS
A DIVISION OF THOMAS NELSON
& ZONDERVAN

WestBow Press books may be ordered through booksellers or by contacting:

WestBow Press
A Division of Thomas Nelson & Zondervan
1663 Liberty Drive
Bloomington, IN 47403
www.westbowpress.com
1 (866) 928-1240

ISBN: 978-1-4908-4487-9 (sc)
ISBN: 978-1-4908-4489-3 (hc)

Library of Congress Control Number: 2014912740

Printed in the United States of America.

WestBow Press rev. date: 10/06/2014

Contents

Introduction

We were sitting in the lobby, waiting for the nurse to come out to call the next patient. The door opened and the nurse emerged.

"Annie Morrow?"

I got up and followed the nurse into the examination room, pushing Mom's wheelchair. The nurse took her blood pressure and temperature, and then said, "The doctor will see you shortly."

A few minutes later the doctor entered the room. "Mrs. Annie, how are you?"

"I feel alright," Mom said, in a soft, sweet, timid voice. I smiled because those were her favorite words. As the doctor started examining her, he asked questions about her medications, treatment by other physicians, previous screenings, results, and appointments. She could answer some, but not all of them. I could only answer a few, based on what I remembered from talking to her. We made it through the appointment okay, but I was a little embarrassed—not just for myself, but for my mom also. I am her daughter, I should have known more about her medical history. I live in Huntsville, Alabama, and she lives in Saint Louis, Missouri, where her doctor appointments are, so I was never there to go with her to her appointments.

After we left the doctor's office, I stopped at a department store and bought a composition book. When we got home, I sat down and went to work. I got all her information together and wrote all her physicians' names, addresses, and phone numbers; all her medications, and the ones she was allergic to; all her insurance information; all her upcoming appointments; information about her illness, conditions, hospital stays, emergency room visits, and anything else I thought the doctor would ask. I started tracking everything about her health. I kept that book with me because I knew she would not be able to keep it up to date.

My mom knew I was keeping track of everything, so when she visited her physicians or other health providers and could not answer a question, their offices would call me to ask about her health, insurance, and other questions. That was okay with me because it was my mom's health!

Even though I was back in Alabama, I still kept track of everything. After each of her appointments, I would ask her everything I needed to update the book. I would sometimes talk to my dad, my brothers, sisters-in-law, family, friends, or whomever went to the doctor with her to find out what I needed to know.

In March, Mom had surgery. Her right leg was amputated. After the surgery, things turned for the worse. Mom was unresponsive, with an endotracheal tube placed down her throat, and fighting for her life. She was in the intensive care unit for a couple of weeks. In the morning, physicians would do their rounds, and whenever they asked me a question about her health and/or her physicians, I would pull out my book. A couple of them commented on the book, saying it was a great idea.

I remember sitting in the intensive care unit with her while the anesthesiologist went over the list of medications that she was allergic to. And, guess what? The list did not include one of the medications it should have had. I would not have known that if I hadn't had my book.

I decided to create *Her Personal Medical Journal* for women like my mom and me to keep track of one of the most important things in life: *our health*.

This is presented in memory of my mom, my love, Annie Lo Morrow, who lost her fight on April 18, 2013.

How to Use This Booklet

Her Personal Medical Journal is created for women like my mom and me—women who visit the doctor's office, but can't remember the answers to simple questions the physicians ask, such as *when was your last menstrual cycle? When was your last mammogram?* Or, *when was your last tetanus shot?* Simple questions that, we cannot answer because we can't remember the exact date, month, name, or location.

Her Personal Medical Journal will allow you to track all of your procedures, surgeries, lists of physicians, medications, and much more.

Use this as *your* personal medical journal. Keep it in a special place, and take it with you every time you go on a doctor visit.

It is up to you to choose what you enter in your booklet. If you don't feel comfortable listing something for fear of losing your booklet, or because you're afraid someone might get their hands on it, then don't. If you cannot keep it in a safe place, **do not put any information in this booklet that you don't want people to know.** Just remember to inform your physicians about any health issues not listed.

There are also several screenings listed in this booklet to help you remember what's important for your health.

PLEASE KEEP THIS BOOKLET IN A SAFE PLACE.

This Personal Medical Journal Belongs to:

Name: _____

Address: _____

City: _____ State: _____ ZIP: _____

Home Phone: _____

Cell Phone: _____

Emergency Contact

Name: _____

Relationship: _____

Address: _____

City: _____ State: _____ ZIP: _____

Home Phone: _____

Cell Phone: _____

Personal

This section is for information about you.

Please list all life habits and hereditary risk factors. These may require preventive screenings before the recommended age.

List all your medical conditions in your *Personal Medical Journal.*

If you have a medical condition that you don't want to list, you can do one of two things:

1. Don't list it! (But remember to inform your physician.)
2. Write *Contact Physician* on the *Medical Condition* line provided, along with physician contact information.

All About Me

Date of Birth: _____

Blood Type: _____

Blood Pressure Range: _____

Weight: _____ Height: _____

Corrected Vision: No ____ Yes ____
       Glasses: _____ Contacts: _____ Both: _____

Lifestyle Habits: _____
_____
_____

Hereditary Risk Factors: _____
_____
_____

Chronic Illness (epilepsy, diabetes, heart disease, etc.): _____
_____
_____

Allergies:
_____
_____
_____

Medical Conditions

Medical Condition: _____

Diagnosed Date: _____

Diagnosed By: _____

Medication for Condition: _____

Dosage: _____ How Often: _____

Medical Condition: _____

Diagnosed Date: _____

Diagnosed By: _____

Medication for Condition: _____

Dosage: _____ How Often: _____

Medical Condition: _____

Diagnosed Date: _____

Diagnosed By: _____

Medication for Condition: _____

Dosage: _____ How Often: _____

Medical Condition: _____

Diagnosed Date: _____

Diagnosed By: _____

Medication for Condition: _____

Dosage: _____ How Often: _____

Medical Condition: _____

Diagnosed Date: _____

Diagnosed By: _____

Medication for Condition: _____

Dosage: _____ How Often: _____

Medical Condition: _____

Diagnosed Date: _____

Diagnosed By: _____

Medication for Condition: _____

Dosage: _____ How Often: _____

Medical Condition: _____

Diagnosed Date: _____

Diagnosed By: _____

Medication for Condition: _____

Dosage: _____ How Often: _____

Medical Condition: _____

Diagnosed Date: _____

Diagnosed By: _____

Medication for Condition: _____

Dosage: _____ How Often: _____

Medical Condition: _____

Diagnosed Date: _____

Diagnosed By: _____

Medication for Condition: _____

Dosage: _____ How Often: _____

Medical Condition: _____

Diagnosed Date: _____

Diagnosed By: _____

Medication for Condition: _____

Dosage: _____ How Often: _____

Medical Condition: _____

Diagnosed Date: _____

Diagnosed By: _____

Medication for Condition: _____

Dosage: _____ How Often: _____

Medical Condition: _____

Diagnosed Date: _____

Diagnosed By: _____

Medication for Condition: _____

Dosage: _____ How Often: _____

Medical Condition: _____

Diagnosed Date: _____

Diagnosed By: _____

Medication for Condition: _____

Dosage: _____ How Often: _____

Medical Condition: _____

Diagnosed Date: _____

Diagnosed By: _____

Medication for Condition: _____

Dosage: _____ How Often: _____

Medical Condition: _____

Diagnosed Date: _____

Diagnosed By: _____

Medication for Condition: _____

Dosage: _____ How Often: _____

Medical Condition: _____

Diagnosed Date: _____

Diagnosed By: _____

Medication for Condition: _____

Dosage: _____ How Often: _____

Medical Condition: _____

Diagnosed Date: _____

Diagnosed By: _____

Medication for Condition: _____

Dosage: _____ How Often: _____

Medical Condition: _____

Diagnosed Date: _____

Diagnosed By: _____

Medication for Condition: _____

Dosage: _____ How Often: _____

Medical Condition: _____

Diagnosed Date: _____

Diagnosed By: _____

Medication for Condition: _____

Dosage: _____ How Often: _____

Medical Condition: _____

Diagnosed Date: _____

Diagnosed By: _____

Medication for Condition: _____

Dosage: _____ How Often: _____

Insurance Information

Please remember to take your insurance card with you on your visits to the physician.

The doctor's office should have your insurance information, and will usually be willing to make a copy to put in your files.

Medical

Company: _____
Contract Number: _____
Group Number: _____
Policy Number: _____
Rx BIN Number: _____
Member Number: _____
PCN Number: _____
Address: _____
City: _____ State: _____ ZIP: _____
Phone Number: (_____) _____

Vision

Company: _____
Member ID: _____
Plan Number: _____
Address: _____
City: _____ State: _____ ZIP: _____
Phone Number: (_____) _____

Dental

Company: _____
Member ID: _____
Plan Number: _____
Address: _____
City: _____ State: _____ ZIP: _____
Phone Number: (_____) _____

Medicaid

Phone Number: (_____) _____
Member Number: _____
Group Number: _____
Bin Number: _____
Benefit Plan: _____
Effective Date: _____

Medicare

Phone Number: (_____) _____
Claim Number: _____

Entitle to: Effective Date
_____ Part A Hospital Insurance   _____
_____ Part B Medical Insurance   _____
_____ Part C Medical Advantage   _____
_____ Part D Prescription Drug Coverage   _____

AARP

Phone Number: (_____) _____
Membership Number: _____

Comments: _____
_____
_____
_____
_____
_____
_____

Comments: _____

_____

_____

_____

_____

_____

_____

_____

_____

_____

_____

_____

_____

_____

_____

_____

_____

_____

_____

_____

_____

_____

_____

_____

_____

_____

_____

_____

Routine Treatments

This section is used to list your routine treatments (e.g., dialysis, chemotherapy, etc.).

Please list the type of treatment, location, day, time, and physician.

If your doctor discontinues a treatment, draw an X across the treatment with a red pen.

Type of Treatment: _____

Location: _____

Address: _____

City: _____ State: _____ ZIP: _____

Phone Number: (___) _____

Days: Mon__ Tue__ Wed__ Thu__ Fri__ Sat__ Sun__

Time: _____   Ordered by: _____

Type of Treatment: _____

Location: _____

Address: _____

City: _____ State: _____ ZIP: _____

Phone Number: (___) _____

Days: Mon__ Tue__ Wed__ Thu__ Fri__ Sat__ Sun__

Time: _____   Ordered by: _____

Type of Treatment: _____

Location: _____

Address: _____

City: _____ State: _____ ZIP: _____

Phone Number: (___) _____

Days: Mon__ Tue__ Wed__ Thu__ Fri__ Sat__ Sun__

Time: _____   Ordered by: _____

Type of Treatment: _____

Location: _____

Address: _____

City: _____ State: _____ ZIP: _____

Phone Number: (___) _____

Days: Mon__ Tue__ Wed__ Thu__ Fri__ Sat__ Sun__

Time: _____   Ordered by: _____

Type of Treatment: _____
Location: _____
Address: _____
City: _____ State: _____ ZIP: _____
Phone Number: (___) _____
Days: Mon__ Tue__ Wed__ Thu__ Fri__ Sat__ Sun__
Time: _____   Ordered by: _____

Type of Treatment: _____
Location: _____
Address: _____
City: _____ State: _____ ZIP: _____
Phone Number: (___) _____
Days: Mon__ Tue__ Wed__ Thu__ Fri__ Sat__ Sun__
Time: _____   Ordered by: _____

Type of Treatment: _____
Location: _____
Address: _____
City: _____ State: _____ ZIP: _____
Phone Number: (___) _____
Days: Mon__ Tue__ Wed__ Thu__ Fri__ Sat__ Sun__
Time: _____   Ordered by: _____

Type of Treatment: _____
Location: _____
Address: _____
City: _____ State: _____ ZIP: _____
Phone Number: (___) _____
Days: Mon__ Tue__ Wed__ Thu__ Fri__ Sat__ Sun__
Time: _____   Ordered by: _____

Type of Treatment: _____
Location: _____
Address: _____
City: _____ State: _____ ZIP: _____
Phone Number: (___) _____
Days: Mon__ Tue__ Wed__ Thu__ Fri__ Sat__ Sun__
Time: _____ Ordered by: _____

Type of Treatment: _____
Location: _____
Address: _____
City: _____ State: _____ ZIP: _____
Phone Number: (___) _____
Days: Mon__ Tue__ Wed__ Thu__ Fri__ Sat__ Sun__
Time: _____ Ordered by: _____

Type of Treatment: _____
Location: _____
Address: _____
City: _____ State: _____ ZIP: _____
Phone Number: (___) _____
Days: Mon__ Tue__ Wed__ Thu__ Fri__ Sat__ Sun__
Time: _____ Ordered by: _____

Type of Treatment: _____
Location: _____
Address: _____
City: _____ State: _____ ZIP: _____
Phone Number: (___) _____
Days: Mon__ Tue__ Wed__ Thu__ Fri__ Sat__ Sun__
Time: _____ Ordered by: _____

Family History

This section is to list your family history and relevant conditions (parents, siblings, grandparents).

Tests and screenings may be indicated based on your family history. Your risk for developing a particular chronic disease may be greater if a close family member has had it.

Mother: _____

Medical Conditions: _____

_____

Cause of Death: _____ Age:_____

Father: _____

Medical Conditions: _____

_____

Cause of Death: _____ Age:_____

Grandmother on Mother's Side: _____

Medical Conditions: _____

_____

Cause of Death: _____ Age:_____

Grandfather on Mother's Side: _____

Medical Conditions: _____

_____

Cause of Death: _____ Age:_____

Grandmother on Father's Side: _____

Medical Conditions: _____

_____

Cause of Death: _____ Age:_____

Grandfather on Father's Side: _____

Medical Conditions: _____

_____

Cause of Death: _____ Age:_____

Sibling: _____

Medical Conditions: _____

_____

Cause of Death: _____ Age:_____

Sibling: _____

Medical Conditions: _____

_____

Cause of Death: _____ Age:_____

Sibling: _____

Medical Conditions: _____

_____

Cause of Death: _____ Age:_____

Sibling: _____

Medical Conditions: _____

_____

Cause of Death: _____ Age:_____

Sibling: _____

Medical Conditions: _____

_____

Cause of Death: _____ Age:_____

Sibling: _____

Medical Conditions: _____

_____

Cause of Death: _____ Age:_____

Sibling: _____
Medical Conditions: _____
_____
Cause of Death: _____ Age:_____

Sibling: _____
Medical Conditions: _____
_____
Cause of Death: _____ Age:_____

Sibling: _____
Medical Conditions: _____
_____
Cause of Death: _____ Age:_____

Sibling: _____
Medical Conditions: _____
_____
Cause of Death: _____ Age:_____

Sibling: _____
Medical Conditions: _____
_____
Cause of Death: _____ Age:_____

Sibling: _____
Medical Conditions: _____
_____
Cause of Death: _____ Age:_____

History of Hospitalizations, Procedures, and Surgeries

This section helps you keep track of previous hospitalizations, procedures, and surgeries.

Your physician may request results from a previous visit to a health care provider.

Date: _____
Hospital: _____
Reason: _____
Notes: _____

_____

Date: _____
Hospital: _____
Reason: _____
Notes: _____

_____

Date: _____
Hospital: _____
Reason: _____
Notes: _____

_____

Date: _____
Hospital: _____
Reason: _____
Notes: _____

_____

Date: _____
Hospital: _____
Reason: _____
Notes: _____

_____

Date: _____
Hospital: _____
Reason: _____
Notes: _____
_____

Date: _____
Hospital: _____
Reason: _____
Notes: _____
_____

Date: _____
Hospital: _____
Reason: _____
Notes: _____
_____

Date: _____
Hospital: _____
Reason: _____
Notes: _____
_____

Date: _____
Hospital: _____
Reason: _____
Notes: _____
_____

Date: _____
Hospital: _____
Reason: _____
Notes: _____
_____

Date: _____
Hospital: _____
Reason: _____
Notes: _____
_____

Date: _____
Hospital: _____
Reason: _____
Notes: _____
_____

Date: _____
Hospital: _____
Reason: _____
Notes: _____
_____

Date: _____
Hospital: _____
Reason: _____
Notes: _____
_____

Date: _____

Hospital: _____

Reason: _____

Notes: _____

_____

Date: _____

Hospital: _____

Reason: _____

Notes: _____

_____

Date: _____

Hospital: _____

Reason: _____

Notes: _____

_____

Date: _____

Hospital: _____

Reason: _____

Notes: _____

_____

Date: _____

Hospital: _____

Reason: _____

Notes: _____

_____

Date: _____
Hospital: _____
Reason: _____
Notes: _____
_____

Date: _____
Hospital: _____
Reason: _____
Notes: _____
_____

Date: _____
Hospital: _____
Reason: _____
Notes: _____
_____

Date: _____
Hospital: _____
Reason: _____
Notes: _____
_____

Date: _____
Hospital: _____
Reason: _____
Notes: _____
_____

Physicians

This section is created to list all physicians, specialists, surgeons, and any other physicians you see.

Enter their name, direct nurse, address, phone number, fax number, exchange number, and office hours.

Dentist

Dentist Name: _____

Address: _____

City: _____ State: _____ ZIP: _____

Phone Number: (_____) _____

Fax Number: (_____) _____

Exchange: (_____) _____

Office Hours: _____

Physicians

Primary Physician: _____

Physician Name: _____

Direct Nurse: _____

Address: _____

City: _____ State: _____ ZIP: _____

Phone Number: (_____) _____

Fax Number: (_____) _____

Exchange: (_____) _____

Office Hours: _____

Physician Type: _____

Physician Name: _____

Direct Nurse: _____

Address: _____

City: _____ State: _____ ZIP: _____

Phone Number: (_____) _____

Fax Number: (_____) _____

Exchange: (_____) _____

Office Hours: _____

Physician Type: _____

Physician Name: _____

Direct Nurse: _____

Address: _____

City: _____ State: _____ ZIP: _____

Phone Number: (_____) _____

Fax Number: (_____) _____

Exchange: (_____) _____

Office Hours: _____

Physician Type: _____

Physician Name: _____

Direct Nurse: _____

Address: _____

City: _____ State: _____ ZIP: _____

Phone Number: (_____) _____

Fax Number: (_____) _____

Exchange: (_____) _____

Office Hours: _____

Physician Type: _____

Physician Name: _____

Direct Nurse: _____

Address: _____

City: _____ State: _____ ZIP: _____

Phone Number: (_____) _____

Fax Number: (_____) _____

Exchange: (_____) _____

Office Hours: _____

Physician Type: _____

Physician Name: _____

Direct Nurse: _____

Address: _____

City: _____ State: _____ ZIP: _____

Phone Number: (____) _____

Fax Number: (____) _____

Exchange: (____) _____

Office Hours: _____

Physician Type: _____

Physician Name: _____

Direct Nurse: _____

Address: _____

City: _____ State: _____ ZIP: _____

Phone Number: (____) _____

Fax Number: (____) _____

Exchange: (____) _____

Office Hours: _____

Physician Type: _____

Physician Name: _____

Direct Nurse: _____

Address: _____

City: _____ State: _____ ZIP: _____

Phone Number: (____) _____

Fax Number: (____) _____

Exchange: (____) _____

Office Hours: _____

Physician Type: _____

Physician Name: _____

Direct Nurse: _____

Address: _____

City: _____ State: _____ ZIP: _____

Phone Number: (____) _____

Fax Number: (____) _____

Exchange: (____) _____

Office Hours: _____

Physician Type: _____

Physician Name: _____

Direct Nurse: _____

Address: _____

City: _____ State: _____ ZIP: _____

Phone Number: (____) _____

Fax Number: (____) _____

Exchange: (____) _____

Office Hours: _____

Physician Type: _____

Physician Name: _____

Direct Nurse: _____

Address: _____

City: _____ State: _____ ZIP: _____

Phone Number: (____) _____

Fax Number: (____) _____

Exchange: (____) _____

Office Hours: _____

Specialists

Specialist Type: _____

Specialist Name: _____

Direct Nurse: _____

Address: _____

City: _____ State: _____ ZIP: _____

Phone Number: (_____) _____

Fax Number: (_____) _____

Exchange: (_____) _____

Office Hours: _____

Specialist Type: _____

Specialist Name: _____

Direct Nurse: _____

Address: _____

City: _____ State: _____ ZIP: _____

Phone Number: (_____) _____

Fax Number: (_____) _____

Exchange: (_____) _____

Office Hours: _____

Specialist Type: _____

Specialist Name: _____

Direct Nurse: _____

Address: _____

City: _____ State: _____ ZIP: _____

Phone Number: (_____) _____

Fax Number: (_____) _____

Exchange: (_____) _____

Office Hours: _____

Specialist Type: _____

Specialist Name: _____

Direct Nurse: _____

Address: _____

City: _____ State: _____ ZIP: _____

Phone Number: (_____) _____

Fax Number: (_____) _____

Exchange: (_____) _____

Office Hours: _____

Specialist Type: _____

Specialist Name: _____

Direct Nurse: _____

Address: _____

City: _____ State: _____ ZIP: _____

Phone Number: (_____) _____

Fax Number: (_____) _____

Exchange: (_____) _____

Office Hours: _____

Specialist Type: _____

Specialist Name: _____

Direct Nurse: _____

Address: _____

City: _____ State: _____ ZIP: _____

Phone Number: (_____) _____

Fax Number: (_____) _____

Exchange: (_____) _____

Office Hours: _____

Surgeons

Surgeon Type: _____

Surgeon Name: _____

Direct Nurse: _____

Address: _____

City: _____ State: _____ ZIP: _____

Phone Number: (_____) _____

Fax Number: (_____) _____

Exchange: (_____) _____

Office Hours: _____

Surgeon Type: _____

Surgeon Name: _____

Direct Nurse: _____

Address: _____

City: _____ State: _____ ZIP: _____

Phone Number: (_____) _____

Fax Number: (_____) _____

Exchange: (_____) _____

Office Hours: _____

Surgeon Type: _____

Surgeon Name: _____

Direct Nurse: _____

Address: _____

City: _____ State: _____ ZIP: _____

Phone Number: (_____) _____

Fax Number: (_____) _____

Exchange: (_____) _____

Office Hours: _____

Surgeon Type: _____

Surgeon Name: _____

Direct Nurse: _____

Address: _____

City: _____ State: _____ ZIP: _____

Phone Number: (_____) _____

Fax Number: (_____) _____

Exchange: (_____) _____

Office Hours: _____

Surgeon Type: _____

Surgeon Name: _____

Direct Nurse: _____

Address: _____

City: _____ State: _____ ZIP: _____

Phone Number: (_____) _____

Fax Number: (_____) _____

Exchange: (_____) _____

Office Hours: _____

Surgeon Type: _____

Surgeon Name: _____

Direct Nurse: _____

Address: _____

City: _____ State: _____ ZIP: _____

Phone Number: (_____) _____

Fax Number: (_____) _____

Exchange: (_____) _____

Office Hours: _____

Additional Information: _____

_____

_____

_____

_____

_____

_____

_____

_____

_____

_____

_____

_____

_____

_____

_____

_____

_____

_____

_____

_____

_____

_____

_____

_____

_____

_____

Med-Center

Please list each medication, who prescribed it, the dosage, and how often you take it.

List *all* medications you are allergic to.

If you are told by a physician to discontinue a medication, *draw an X across the medication with a red pen*, and list it on the *Discontinued Medications* page, along with the name of the physician, date, and reason for discontinuing the medication.

Stop! I am allergic to:

Medication: _____

Side Effects: _____

_____

Medication: _____

Side Effects: _____

_____

Medication: _____

Side Effects: _____

_____

Medication: _____

Side Effects: _____

_____

Medication: _____

Side Effects: _____

_____

Medication: _____

Side Effects: _____

_____

Medication: _____

Side Effects: _____

_____

Medication: _____
Side Effects: _____

_____

Medication: _____
Side Effects: _____

_____

Medication: _____
Side Effects: _____

_____

Medication: _____
Side Effects: _____

_____

Medication: _____
Side Effects: _____

_____

Medication: _____
Side Effects: _____

_____

Medication: _____
Side Effects: _____

_____

Medication: _____
Side Effects: _____

_____

Prescribed Medications

Medication: _____

Reason for Medication: _____

Dosage: _____ How Often: _____

Date Prescribed: _____

Prescribed By: _____

Physician Phone Number: (_____) _____

Medication: _____

Reason for Medication: _____

Dosage: _____ How Often: _____

Date Prescribed: _____

Prescribed By: _____

Physician Phone Number: (_____) _____

Medication: _____

Reason for Medication: _____

Dosage: _____ How Often: _____

Date Prescribed: _____

Prescribed By: _____

Physician Phone Number: (_____) _____

Medication: _____

Reason for Medication: _____

Dosage: _____ How Often: _____

Date Prescribed: _____

Prescribed By: _____

Physician Phone Number: (_____) _____

Medication: _____

Reason for Medication: _____

Dosage: _____ How Often: _____

Date Prescribed: _____

Prescribed By: _____

Physician Phone Number: (____) _____

Medication: _____

Reason for Medication: _____

Dosage: _____ How Often: _____

Date Prescribed: _____

Prescribed By: _____

Physician Phone Number: (____) _____

Medication: _____

Reason for Medication: _____

Dosage: _____ How Often: _____

Date Prescribed: _____

Prescribed By: _____

Physician Phone Number: (____) _____

Medication: _____

Reason for Medication: _____

Dosage: _____ How Often: _____

Date Prescribed: _____

Prescribed By: _____

Physician Phone Number: (____) _____

Medication: _____

Reason for Medication: _____

Dosage: _____ How Often: _____

Date Prescribed: _____

Prescribed By: _____

Physician Phone Number: (____) _____

Medication: _____

Reason for Medication: _____

Dosage: _____ How Often: _____

Date Prescribed: _____

Prescribed By: _____

Physician Phone Number: (____) _____

Medication: _____

Reason for Medication: _____

Dosage: _____ How Often: _____

Date Prescribed: _____

Prescribed By: _____

Physician Phone Number: (____) _____

Medication: _____

Reason for Medication: _____

Dosage: _____ How Often: _____

Date Prescribed: _____

Prescribed By: _____

Physician Phone Number: (____) _____

Medication: _____

Reason for Medication: _____

Dosage: _____ How Often: _____

Date Prescribed: _____

Prescribed By: _____

Physician Phone Number: (_____) _____

Medication: _____

Reason for Medication: _____

Dosage: _____ How Often: _____

Date Prescribed: _____

Prescribed By: _____

Physician Phone Number: (_____) _____

Medication: _____

Reason for Medication: _____

Dosage: _____ How Often: _____

Date Prescribed: _____

Prescribed By: _____

Physician Phone Number: (_____) _____

Medication: _____

Reason for Medication: _____

Dosage: _____ How Often: _____

Date Prescribed: _____

Prescribed By: _____

Physician Phone Number: (_____) _____

Medication: _____

Reason for Medication: _____

Dosage: _____ How Often: _____

Date Prescribed: _____

Prescribed By: _____

Physician Phone Number: (_____) _____

Medication: _____

Reason for Medication: _____

Dosage: _____ How Often: _____

Date Prescribed: _____

Prescribed By: _____

Physician Phone Number: (_____) _____

Medication: _____

Reason for Medication: _____

Dosage: _____ How Often: _____

Date Prescribed: _____

Prescribed By: _____

Physician Phone Number: (_____) _____

Medication: _____

Reason for Medication: _____

Dosage: _____ How Often: _____

Date Prescribed: _____

Prescribed By: _____

Physician Phone Number: (_____) _____

Medication: _____

Reason for Medication: _____

Dosage: _____ How Often: _____

Date Prescribed: _____

Prescribed By: _____

Physician Phone Number: (_____) _____

Medication: _____

Reason for Medication: _____

Dosage: _____ How Often: _____

Date Prescribed: _____

Prescribed By: _____

Physician Phone Number: (_____) _____

Medication: _____

Reason for Medication: _____

Dosage: _____ How Often: _____

Date Prescribed: _____

Prescribed By: _____

Physician Phone Number: (_____) _____

Medication: _____

Reason for Medication: _____

Dosage: _____ How Often: _____

Date Prescribed: _____

Prescribed By: _____

Physician Phone Number: (_____) _____

Medication: _____

Reason for Medication: _____

Dosage: _____ How Often: _____

Date Prescribed: _____

Prescribed By: _____

Physician Phone Number: (_____) _____

Medication: _____

Reason for Medication: _____

Dosage: _____ How Often: _____

Date Prescribed: _____

Prescribed By: _____

Physician Phone Number: (_____) _____

Medication: _____

Reason for Medication: _____

Dosage: _____ How Often: _____

Date Prescribed: _____

Prescribed By: _____

Physician Phone Number: (_____) _____

Medication: _____

Reason for Medication: _____

Dosage: _____ How Often: _____

Date Prescribed: _____

Prescribed By: _____

Physician Phone Number: (_____) _____

Medication: _____

Reason for Medication: _____

Dosage: _____ How Often: _____

Date Prescribed: _____

Prescribed By: _____

Physician Phone Number: (____) _____

Medication: _____

Reason for Medication: _____

Dosage: _____ How Often: _____

Date Prescribed: _____

Prescribed By: _____

Physician Phone Number: (____) _____

Medication: _____

Reason for Medication: _____

Dosage: _____ How Often: _____

Date Prescribed: _____

Prescribed By: _____

Physician Phone Number: (____) _____

Medication: _____

Reason for Medication: _____

Dosage: _____ How Often: _____

Date Prescribed: _____

Prescribed By: _____

Physician Phone Number: (____) _____

Over-the-Counter Supplements

Supplement: _____
Date Started: _____ Dosage:_____ mg: _____

Supplement: _____
Date Started: _____ Dosage:_____ mg: _____

Supplement: _____
Date Started: _____ Dosage:_____ mg: _____

Supplement: _____
Date Started: _____ Dosage:_____ mg: _____

Supplement: _____
Date Started: _____ Dosage:_____ mg: _____

Supplement: _____
Date Started: _____ Dosage:_____ mg: _____

Supplement: _____
Date Started: _____ Dosage:_____ mg: _____

Supplement: _____
Date Started: _____ Dosage:_____ mg: _____

Supplement: _____
Date Started: _____ Dosage:_____ mg: _____

Supplement: _____
Date Started: _____ Dosage:_____ mg: _____

Supplement: _____
Date Started: _____ Dosage:_____ mg: _____

Supplement: _____

Date Started: _____ Dosage:_____ mg: _____

Supplement: _____

Date Started: _____ Dosage:_____ mg: _____

Supplement: _____

Date Started: _____ Dosage:_____ mg: _____

Supplement: _____

Date Started: _____ Dosage:_____ mg: _____

Supplement: _____

Date Started: _____ Dosage:_____ mg: _____

Supplement: _____

Date Started: _____ Dosage:_____ mg: _____

Supplement: _____

Date Started: _____ Dosage:_____ mg: _____

Supplement: _____

Date Started: _____ Dosage:_____ mg: _____

Supplement: _____

Date Started: _____ Dosage:_____ mg: _____

Supplement: _____

Date Started: _____ Dosage:_____ mg: _____

Supplement: _____

Date Started: _____ Dosage:_____ mg: _____

Discontinued Medications

Discontinued Medication: _____

Discontinued By: _____

Reason for Discontinuing: _____

_____

Discontinued Date: _____

Discontinued Medication: _____

Discontinued By: _____

Reason for Discontinuing: _____

_____

Discontinued Date: _____

Discontinued Medication: _____

Discontinued By: _____

Reason for Discontinuing: _____

_____

Discontinued Date: _____

Discontinued Medication: _____

Discontinued By: _____

Reason for Discontinuing: _____

_____

Discontinued Date: _____

Discontinued Medication: _____

Discontinued By: _____

Reason for Discontinuing: _____

_____

Discontinued Date: _____

Discontinued Medication: _____

Discontinued By: _____

Reason for Discontinuing: _____

_____

Discontinued Date: _____

Discontinued Medication: _____

Discontinued By: _____

Reason for Discontinuing: _____

_____

Discontinued Date: _____

Discontinued Medication: _____

Discontinued By: _____

Reason for Discontinuing: _____

_____

Discontinued Date: _____

Discontinued Medication: _____

Discontinued By: _____

Reason for Discontinuing: _____

_____

Discontinued Date: _____

Discontinued Medication: _____

Discontinued By: _____

Reason for Discontinuing: _____

_____

Discontinued Date: _____

Discontinued Medication: _____

Discontinued By: _____

Reason for Discontinuing: _____

_____

Discontinued Date: _____

Discontinued Medication: _____

Discontinued By: _____

Reason for Discontinuing: _____

_____

Discontinued Date: _____

Discontinued Medication: _____

Discontinued By: _____

Reason for Discontinuing: _____

_____

Discontinued Date: _____

Discontinued Medication: _____

Discontinued By: _____

Reason for Discontinuing: _____

_____

Discontinued Date: _____

Discontinued Medication: _____

Discontinued By: _____

Reason for Discontinuing: _____

_____

Discontinued Date: _____

Discontinued Medication: _____

Discontinued By: _____

Reason for Discontinuing: _____

_____

Discontinued Date: _____

Discontinued Medication: _____

Discontinued By: _____

Reason for Discontinuing: _____

_____

Discontinued Date: _____

Discontinued Medication: _____

Discontinued By: _____

Reason for Discontinuing: _____

_____

Discontinued Date: _____

Discontinued Medication: _____

Discontinued By: _____

Reason for Discontinuing: _____

_____

Discontinued Date: _____

Discontinued Medication: _____

Discontinued By: _____

Reason for Discontinuing: _____

_____

Discontinued Date: _____

Discontinued Medication: _____
Discontinued By: _____
Reason for Discontinuing: _____

_____

Discontinued Date: _____

Discontinued Medication: _____
Discontinued By: _____
Reason for Discontinuing: _____

_____

Discontinued Date: _____

Discontinued Medication: _____
Discontinued By: _____
Reason for Discontinuing: _____

_____

Discontinued Date: _____

Discontinued Medication: _____
Discontinued By: _____
Reason for Discontinuing: _____

_____

Discontinued Date: _____

Discontinued Medication: _____
Discontinued By: _____
Reason for Discontinuing: _____

_____

Discontinued Date: _____

Pharmacy

Using *only one* pharmacy helps reduce the chances of bad drug interactions or duplications.

Your pharmacy can check your file and tell you about potential problems with the other medications you are taking. This is only possible if you fill your prescriptions at *one* pharmacy. List only one pharmacy and other locations for the same pharmacy. It may be in the same state or another state.

Pharmacy Name _____

First Location
Address: _____
City:_____ State:_____ ZIP:_____
Phone Number: (____) _____
Pharmacy Hours: _____

Second Location
Address: _____
City:_____ State:_____ ZIP:_____
Phone Number: (____) _____
Pharmacy Hours: _____

Third Location
Address: _____
City:_____ State:_____ ZIP:_____
Phone Number: (____) _____
Pharmacy Hours: _____

Fourth Location
Address: _____
City:_____ State:_____ ZIP:_____
Phone Number: (____) _____
Pharmacy Hours: _____

When Is My Next Appointment?

This section is used to track your next appointment for dental and other physician visits.

You can also track all your procedures and surgeries.

Dental

Next Appointment Date: _____ Time: _____
Treatment: _____
_____

Next Appointment Date: _____ Time: _____
Treatment: _____
_____

Next Appointment Date: _____ Time: _____
Treatment: _____
_____

Next Appointment Date: _____ Time: _____
Treatment: _____
_____

Next Appointment Date: _____ Time: _____
Treatment: _____
_____

Next Appointment Date: _____ Time: _____
Treatment: _____
_____

Next Appointment Date: _____ Time: _____
Treatment: _____
_____

Next Appointment Date: _____ Time: _____
Treatment: _____
_____

Next Appointment Date: _____ Time: _____
Treatment: _____

_____

Next Appointment Date: _____ Time: _____
Treatment: _____

_____

Next Appointment Date: _____ Time: _____
Treatment: _____

_____

Next Appointment Date: _____ Time: _____
Treatment: _____

_____

Next Appointment Date: _____ Time: _____
Treatment: _____

_____

Next Appointment Date: _____ Time: _____
Treatment: _____

_____

Next Appointment Date: _____ Time: _____
Treatment: _____

_____

Next Appointment Date: _____ Time: _____
Treatment: _____

_____

Physicians

Appointment With: _____

Date: _____ Time:_____

Special Notes: _____

_____

Appointment With: _____

Date: _____ Time:_____

Special Notes: _____

_____

Appointment With: _____

Date: _____ Time:_____

Special Notes: _____

_____

Appointment With: _____

Date: _____ Time:_____

Special Notes: _____

_____

Appointment With: _____

Date: _____ Time:_____

Special Notes: _____

_____

Appointment With: _____

Date: _____ Time:_____

Special Notes: _____

_____

Appointment With: _____
Date: _____ Time: _____
Special Notes: _____
_____

Appointment With: _____
Date: _____ Time: _____
Special Notes: _____
_____

Appointment With: _____
Date: _____ Time: _____
Special Notes: _____
_____

Appointment With: _____
Date: _____ Time: _____
Special Notes: _____
_____

Appointment With: _____
Date: _____ Time: _____
Special Notes: _____
_____

Appointment With: _____
Date: _____ Time: _____
Special Notes: _____
_____

Appointment With: _____

Date: _____ Time: _____

Special Notes: _____

_____

Appointment With: _____

Date: _____ Time: _____

Special Notes: _____

_____

Appointment With: _____

Date: _____ Time: _____

Special Notes: _____

_____

Appointment With: _____

Date: _____ Time: _____

Special Notes: _____

_____

Appointment With: _____

Date: _____ Time: _____

Special Notes: _____

_____

Appointment With: _____

Date: _____ Time: _____

Special Notes: _____

_____

Appointment With: _____

Date: _____ Time:_____

Special Notes: _____

_____

Appointment With: _____

Date: _____ Time:_____

Special Notes: _____

_____

Appointment With: _____

Date: _____ Time:_____

Special Notes: _____

_____

Appointment With: _____

Date: _____ Time:_____

Special Notes: _____

_____

Appointment With: _____

Date: _____ Time:_____

Special Notes: _____

_____

Appointment With: _____

Date: _____ Time:_____

Special Notes: _____

_____

Appointment With: _____
Date: _____ Time:_____
Special Notes: _____
_____

Appointment With: _____
Date: _____ Time:_____
Special Notes: _____
_____

Appointment With: _____
Date: _____ Time:_____
Special Notes: _____
_____

Appointment With: _____
Date: _____ Time:_____
Special Notes: _____
_____

Appointment With: _____
Date: _____ Time:_____
Special Notes: _____
_____

Appointment With: _____
Date: _____ Time:_____
Special Notes: _____
_____

Appointment With: _____

Date: _____ Time:_____

Special Notes: _____

_____

Appointment With: _____

Date: _____ Time:_____

Special Notes: _____

_____

Appointment With: _____

Date: _____ Time:_____

Special Notes: _____

_____

Appointment With: _____

Date: _____ Time:_____

Special Notes: _____

_____

Appointment With: _____

Date: _____ Time:_____

Special Notes: _____

_____

Appointment With: _____

Date: _____ Time:_____

Special Notes: _____

_____

Appointment With: _____

Date: _____ Time:_____

Special Notes: _____

_____

Appointment With: _____

Date: _____ Time:_____

Special Notes: _____

_____

Appointment With: _____

Date: _____ Time:_____

Special Notes: _____

_____

Appointment With: _____

Date: _____ Time:_____

Special Notes: _____

_____

Appointment With: _____

Date: _____ Time:_____

Special Notes: _____

_____

Appointment With: _____

Date: _____ Time:_____

Special Notes: _____

_____

Appointment With: _____

Date: _____ Time:_____

Special Notes: _____

_____

Appointment With: _____

Date: _____ Time:_____

Special Notes: _____

_____

Appointment With: _____

Date: _____ Time:_____

Special Notes: _____

_____

Appointment With: _____

Date: _____ Time:_____

Special Notes: _____

_____

Appointment With: _____

Date: _____ Time:_____

Special Notes: _____

_____

Appointment With: _____

Date: _____ Time:_____

Special Notes: _____

_____

Appointment With: _____

Date: _____ Time: _____

Special Notes: _____

_____

Appointment With: _____

Date: _____ Time: _____

Special Notes: _____

_____

Appointment With: _____

Date: _____ Time: _____

Special Notes: _____

_____

Appointment With: _____

Date: _____ Time: _____

Special Notes: _____

_____

Appointment With: _____

Date: _____ Time: _____

Special Notes: _____

_____

Appointment With: _____

Date: _____ Time: _____

Special Notes: _____

_____

Procedures

Type of Procedure: _____

Date of Procedure: _____ Time:_____

Who will perform the procedure? _____

Reason for procedure: _____

Where will the procedure be performed? _____

Address: _____

City: _____ State:_____ ZIP: _____

Phone Number: (____) _____

Follow-up: _____

Notes: _____

_____

_____

_____

Type of Procedure: _____

Date of Procedure: _____ Time:_____

Who will perform the procedure? _____

Reason for procedure: _____

Where will the procedure be performed? _____

Address: _____

City: _____ State:_____ ZIP: _____

Phone Number: (____) _____

Follow-up: _____

Notes: _____

_____

_____

_____

Type of Procedure: _____

Date of Procedure: _____ Time:_____

Who will perform the procedure? _____

Reason for procedure: _____

Where will the procedure be performed? _____

Address: _____

City: _____ State:_____ ZIP: _____

Phone Number: (_____) _____

Follow-up: _____

Notes: _____

_____

_____

_____

Type of Procedure: _____

Date of Procedure: _____ Time:_____

Who will perform the procedure? _____

Reason for procedure: _____

Where will the procedure be performed? _____

Address: _____

City: _____ State:_____ ZIP: _____

Phone Number: (_____) _____

Follow-up: _____

Notes: _____

_____

_____

_____

Type of Procedure: _____

Date of Procedure: _____ Time:_____

Who will perform the procedure? _____

Reason for procedure: _____

Where will the procedure be performed? _____

Address: _____

City: _____ State:_____ ZIP: _____

Phone Number: (_____) _____

Follow-up: _____

Notes: _____

_____

_____

_____

Type of Procedure: _____

Date of Procedure: _____ Time:_____

Who will perform the procedure? _____

Reason for procedure: _____

Where will the procedure be performed? _____

Address: _____

City: _____ State:_____ ZIP: _____

Phone Number: (_____) _____

Follow-up: _____

Notes: _____

_____

_____

_____

Type of Procedure: _____

Date of Procedure: _____ Time: _____

Who will perform the procedure? _____

Reason for procedure: _____

Where will the procedure be performed? _____

Address: _____

City: _____ State: _____ ZIP: _____

Phone Number: (____) _____

Follow-up: _____

Notes: _____

_____

_____

_____

Type of Procedure: _____

Date of Procedure: _____ Time: _____

Who will perform the procedure? _____

Reason for procedure: _____

Where will the procedure be performed? _____

Address: _____

City: _____ State: _____ ZIP: _____

Phone Number: (____) _____

Follow-up: _____

Notes: _____

_____

_____

_____

Surgeries

Type of Surgery: _____

Date of surgery: _____ Time:_____

Surgeon Name: _____

Address: _____

City: _____ State:_____ ZIP: _____

Phone Number: (____) _____

Where will the surgery be performed? _____

Address: _____

City: _____ State:_____ ZIP: _____

Phone Number: (____) _____

Reason for surgery: _____

Rehabilitation: _____

Notes: _____

_____

Type of Surgery: _____

Date of surgery: _____ Time:_____

Surgeon Name: _____

Address: _____

City: _____ State:_____ ZIP: _____

Phone Number: (____) _____

Where will the surgery be performed? _____

Address: _____

City: _____ State:_____ ZIP: _____

Phone Number: (____) _____

Reason for surgery: _____

Rehabilitation: _____

Notes: _____

_____

Type of Surgery: _____

Date of surgery: _____ Time:_____

Surgeon Name: _____

Address: _____

City: _____ State:_____ ZIP: _____

Phone Number: (____) _____

Where will the surgery be performed? _____

Address: _____

City: _____ State:_____ ZIP: _____

Phone Number: (____) _____

Reason for surgery: _____

Rehabilitation: _____

Notes: _____

_____

Type of Surgery: _____

Date of surgery: _____ Time:_____

Surgeon Name: _____

Address: _____

City: _____ State:_____ ZIP: _____

Phone Number: (____) _____

Where will the surgery be performed? _____

Address: _____

City: _____ State:_____ ZIP: _____

Phone Number: (____) _____

Reason for surgery: _____

Rehabilitation: _____

Notes: _____

_____

Type of Surgery: _____

Date of surgery: _____ Time:_____

Surgeon Name: _____

Address: _____

City: _____ State:_____ ZIP: _____

Phone Number: (____) _____

Where will the surgery be performed? _____

Address: _____

City: _____ State:_____ ZIP: _____

Phone Number: (____) _____

Reason for surgery: _____

Rehabilitation: _____

Notes: _____

_____

Type of Surgery: _____

Date of surgery: _____ Time:_____

Surgeon Name: _____

Address: _____

City: _____ State:_____ ZIP: _____

Phone Number: (____) _____

Where will the surgery be performed? _____

Address: _____

City: _____ State:_____ ZIP: _____

Phone Number: (____) _____

Reason for surgery: _____

Rehabilitation: _____

Notes: _____

_____

Type of Surgery: _____

Date of surgery: _____ Time:_____

Surgeon Name: _____

Address: _____

City: _____ State:_____ ZIP: _____

Phone Number: (_____) _____

Where will the surgery be performed? _____

Address: _____

City: _____ State:_____ ZIP: _____

Phone Number: (_____) _____

Reason for surgery: _____

Rehabilitation: _____

Notes: _____

_____

Type of Surgery: _____

Date of surgery: _____ Time:_____

Surgeon Name: _____

Address: _____

City: _____ State:_____ ZIP: _____

Phone Number: (_____) _____

Where will the surgery be performed? _____

Address: _____

City: _____ State:_____ ZIP: _____

Phone Number: (_____) _____

Reason for surgery: _____

Rehabilitation: _____

Notes: _____

_____

Emergency Room Visits

This section is used to list your emergency room visits and reason for each visit.

Please list the date, hospital, reason, and any other pertinent information.

Date: _____
Hospital: _____
Reason: _____
Comments: _____

Date: _____
Hospital: _____
Reason: _____
Comments: _____

Date: _____
Hospital: _____
Reason: _____
Comments: _____

Date: _____
Hospital: _____
Reason: _____
Comments: _____

Date: _____
Hospital: _____
Reason: _____
Comments: _____

Date: _____
Hospital: _____
Reason: _____
Comments: _____

Date: _____

Hospital: _____

Reason: _____

Comments: _____

Date: _____

Hospital: _____

Reason: _____

Comments: _____

Date: _____

Hospital: _____

Reason: _____

Comments: _____

Date: _____

Hospital: _____

Reason: _____

Comments: _____

Date: _____

Hospital: _____

Reason: _____

Comments: _____

Date: _____

Hospital: _____

Reason: _____

Comments: _____

Date: _____

Hospital: _____

Reason: _____

Comments: _____

Date: _____

Hospital: _____

Reason: _____

Comments: _____

Date: _____

Hospital: _____

Reason: _____

Comments: _____

Date: _____

Hospital: _____

Reason: _____

Comments: _____

Date: _____

Hospital: _____

Reason: _____

Comments: _____

Date: _____

Hospital: _____

Reason: _____

Comments: _____

Making Appointments

Do not get this confused with the *next appointment*! Use this section when you are not feeling well and need to make an appointment to see your physician.

Physician: _____

Reason: _____

When did it start? _____

Do you know what caused it?_____

Questions for Physician: _____

_____

_____

Physician: _____

Reason: _____

When did it start? _____

Do you know what caused it?_____

Questions for Physician: _____

_____

_____

Physician: _____

Reason: _____

When did it start? _____

Do you know what caused it?_____

Questions for Physician: _____

_____

_____

Physician: _____

Reason: _____

When did it start? _____

Do you know what caused it?_____

Questions for Physician: _____

_____

_____

Physician: _____
Reason: _____
When did it start? _____
Do you know what caused it?_____
Questions for Physician: _____

_____

_____

Physician: _____
Reason: _____
When did it start? _____
Do you know what caused it?_____
Questions for Physician: _____

_____

_____

Physician: _____
Reason: _____
When did it start? _____
Do you know what caused it?_____
Questions for Physician: _____

_____

_____

Physician: _____
Reason: _____
When did it start? _____
Do you know what caused it?_____
Questions for Physician: _____

_____

_____

Physician: _____

Reason: _____

When did it start? _____

Do you know what caused it?_____

Questions for Physician: _____

_____

_____

Physician: _____

Reason: _____

When did it start? _____

Do you know what caused it?_____

Questions for Physician: _____

_____

_____

Physician: _____

Reason: _____

When did it start? _____

Do you know what caused it?_____

Questions for Physician: _____

_____

_____

Physician: _____

Reason: _____

When did it start? _____

Do you know what caused it?_____

Questions for Physician: _____

_____

_____

Physician: _____

Reason: _____

When did it start? _____

Do you know what caused it?_____

Questions for Physician: _____

_____

_____

Physician: _____

Reason: _____

When did it start? _____

Do you know what caused it?_____

Questions for Physician: _____

_____

_____

Physician: _____

Reason: _____

When did it start? _____

Do you know what caused it?_____

Questions for Physician: _____

_____

_____

Physician: _____

Reason: _____

When did it start? _____

Do you know what caused it?_____

Questions for Physician: _____

_____

_____

Physician: _____

Reason: _____

When did it start? _____

Do you know what caused it?_____

Questions for Physician: _____

_____

_____

Physician: _____

Reason: _____

When did it start? _____

Do you know what caused it?_____

Questions for Physician: _____

_____

_____

Physician: _____

Reason: _____

When did it start? _____

Do you know what caused it?_____

Questions for Physician: _____

_____

_____

Physician: _____

Reason: _____

When did it start? _____

Do you know what caused it?_____

Questions for Physician: _____

_____

_____

Physician: _____

Reason: _____

When did it start? _____

Do you know what caused it?_____

Questions for Physician: _____

_____

_____

Physician: _____

Reason: _____

When did it start? _____

Do you know what caused it?_____

Questions for Physician: _____

_____

_____

Physician: _____

Reason: _____

When did it start? _____

Do you know what caused it?_____

Questions for Physician: _____

_____

_____

Physician: _____

Reason: _____

When did it start? _____

Do you know what caused it?_____

Questions for Physician: _____

_____

_____

Physician: _____

Reason: _____

When did it start? _____

Do you know what caused it?_____

Questions for Physician: _____

_____

_____

Physician: _____

Reason: _____

When did it start? _____

Do you know what caused it?_____

Questions for Physician: _____

_____

_____

Physician: _____

Reason: _____

When did it start? _____

Do you know what caused it?_____

Questions for Physician: _____

_____

_____

Physician: _____

Reason: _____

When did it start? _____

Do you know what caused it?_____

Questions for Physician: _____

_____

_____

Tracking

You may track your menstrual cycle, your weight and height, if needed, and any type of shots you've received.

Menstrual

I started my menstrual cycle at the age of: _____
My cycle usually last _____ days

Start Date   **End Date**

_____   _____
_____   _____
_____   _____
_____   _____
_____   _____
_____   _____
_____   _____
_____   _____
_____   _____
_____   _____
_____   _____
_____   _____
_____   _____
_____   _____
_____   _____
_____   _____
_____   _____
_____   _____
_____   _____
_____   _____
_____   _____
_____   _____
_____   _____
_____   _____
_____   _____

Start Date   **End Date**

_____   _____

_____   _____

_____   _____

_____   _____

_____   _____

_____   _____

_____   _____

_____   _____

_____   _____

_____   _____

_____   _____

_____   _____

_____   _____

_____   _____

_____   _____

_____   _____

_____   _____

_____   _____

_____   _____

_____   _____

_____   _____

_____   _____

_____   _____

_____   _____

_____   _____

_____   _____

_____   _____

_____   _____

_____   _____

_____   _____

Start Date   **End Date**

_____   _____

_____   _____

_____   _____

_____   _____

_____   _____

_____   _____

_____   _____

_____   _____

_____   _____

_____   _____

_____   _____

_____   _____

_____   _____

_____   _____

_____   _____

_____   _____

_____   _____

_____   _____

_____   _____

_____   _____

_____   _____

_____   _____

_____   _____

_____   _____

_____   _____

Height and Weight

Date: _____ Height: _____ Weight:_____
Date: _____ Height: _____ Weight:_____
Date: _____ Height: _____ Weight:_____
Date: _____ Height: _____ Weight:_____
Date: _____ Height: _____ Weight:_____
Date: _____ Height: _____ Weight:_____
Date: _____ Height: _____ Weight:_____
Date: _____ Height: _____ Weight:_____
Date: _____ Height: _____ Weight:_____
Date: _____ Height: _____ Weight:_____
Date: _____ Height: _____ Weight:_____
Date: _____ Height: _____ Weight:_____
Date: _____ Height: _____ Weight:_____
Date: _____ Height: _____ Weight:_____
Date: _____ Height: _____ Weight:_____
Date: _____ Height: _____ Weight:_____
Date: _____ Height: _____ Weight:_____
Date: _____ Height: _____ Weight:_____
Date: _____ Height: _____ Weight:_____
Date: _____ Height: _____ Weight:_____
Date: _____ Height: _____ Weight:_____
Date: _____ Height: _____ Weight:_____
Date: _____ Height: _____ Weight:_____
Date: _____ Height: _____ Weight:_____
Date: _____ Height: _____ Weight:_____
Date: _____ Height: _____ Weight:_____
Date: _____ Height: _____ Weight:_____
Date: _____ Height: _____ Weight:_____
Date: _____ Height: _____ Weight:_____
Date: _____ Height: _____ Weight:_____

Shots Tracker

Date: _____
Type: _____

Date: _____
Type: _____

Date: _____
Type: _____

Date: _____
Type: _____

Date: _____
Type: _____

Date: _____
Type: _____

Date: _____
Type: _____

Date: _____
Type: _____

Date: _____
Type: _____

Date: _____
Type: _____

Date: _____
Type: _____

Screening Tests for Women

This is a list of the common screenings that are important for women.

Please check with your primary physician for other screenings.

Your doctor or nurse will personalize the timing of the screening tests you need, based on many factors.

You may log other tests under *Other Screenings and/or Tests.*

Blood Pressure Test

A blood pressure test measures the pressure in your arteries as your heart pumps. This is one of the most important screenings because high blood pressure often has no symptoms, so it can't be detected without being measured. High blood pressure greatly increases your risk of heart disease and stroke.

Systolic (Sys) Diastolic (Dia) Heart Rate (HR)

Date: _____ Time:_____ Sys:____ Dia:____ HR: _____

Date: _____ Time:_____ Sys:____ Dia:____ HR: _____

Date: _____ Time:_____ Sys:____ Dia:____ HR: _____

Date: _____ Time:_____ Sys:____ Dia:____ HR: _____

Date: _____ Time:_____ Sys:____ Dia:____ HR: _____

Date: _____ Time:_____ Sys:____ Dia:____ HR: _____

Date: _____ Time:_____ Sys:____ Dia:____ HR: _____

Date: _____ Time:_____ Sys:____ Dia:____ HR: _____

Date: _____ Time:_____ Sys:____ Dia:____ HR: _____

Date: _____ Time:_____ Sys:____ Dia:____ HR: _____

Date: _____ Time:_____ Sys:____ Dia:____ HR: _____

Date: _____ Time:_____ Sys:____ Dia:____ HR: _____

Date: _____ Time:_____ Sys:____ Dia:____ HR: _____

Date: _____ Time:_____ Sys:____ Dia:____ HR: _____

Date: _____ Time:_____ Sys:____ Dia:____ HR: _____

Date: _____ Time:_____ Sys:____ Dia:____ HR: _____

Date: _____ Time:_____ Sys:____ Dia:____ HR: _____

Date: _____ Time:_____ Sys:____ Dia:____ HR: _____

Date: _____ Time:_____ Sys:____ Dia:____ HR: _____

Date: _____ Time:_____ Sys:____ Dia:____ HR: _____

Date: _____ Time:_____ Sys:____ Dia:____ HR: _____

Bone Mineral Density

A bone density test measures your bone health. It determines if you have osteoporosis—a disease that causes bones to become more fragile and more likely to break.

Test Date: _____
Place of Service: _____
Address: _____
City:_____ State: _____ ZIP:_____
Phone Number: (____) _____
Ordered By: _____

Test Date: _____
Place of Service: _____
Address: _____
City:_____ State: _____ ZIP:_____
Phone Number: (____) _____
Ordered By: _____

Test Date: _____
Place of Service: _____
Address: _____
City:_____ State: _____ ZIP:_____
Phone Number: (____) _____

Ordered By: _____

Mammogram

A mammogram is an X-ray image of your breast used to screen for breast cancer.

Date: _____
Type: _____
Place of Service: _____
Address: _____
City: _____ State: _____ ZIP: _____
Phone Number: (___) _____
Ultrasound Needed? Yes__ No__ Right__ Left__ Both__

Date: _____
Type: _____
Place of Service: _____
Address: _____
City: _____ State: _____ ZIP: _____
Phone Number: (___) _____
Ultrasound Needed? Yes__ No__ Right__ Left__ Both__

Date: _____
Type: _____
Place of Service: _____
Address: _____
City: _____ State: _____ ZIP: _____
Phone Number: (___) _____
Ultrasound Needed? Yes__ No__ Right__ Left__ Both__

Date: _____
Type: _____
Place of Service: _____
Address: _____
City: _____ State: _____ ZIP: _____
Phone Number: (___) _____
Ultrasound Needed? Yes__ No__ Right__ Left__ Both__

Date: _____
Type: _____
Place of Service: _____
Address: _____
City: _____ State: _____ ZIP: _____
Phone Number: (___) _____
Ultrasound Needed? Yes__ No__ Right__ Left__ Both__

Date: _____
Type: _____
Place of Service: _____
Address: _____
City: _____ State: _____ ZIP: _____
Phone Number: (___) _____
Ultrasound Needed? Yes__ No__ Right__ Left__ Both__

Date: _____
Type: _____
Place of Service: _____
Address: _____
City: _____ State: _____ ZIP: _____
Phone Number: (___) _____
Ultrasound Needed? Yes__ No__ Right__ Left__ Both__

Date: _____

Type: _____

Place of Service: _____

Address: _____

City: _____ State: _____ ZIP: _____

Phone Number: (___) _____

Ultrasound Needed? Yes__ No__ Right__ Left__ Both__

Date: _____

Type: _____

Place of Service: _____

Address: _____

City: _____ State: _____ ZIP: _____

Phone Number: (___) _____

Ultrasound Needed? Yes__ No__ Right__ Left__ Both__

Date: _____

Type: _____

Place of Service: _____

Address: _____

City: _____ State: _____ ZIP: _____

Phone Number: (___) _____

Ultrasound Needed? Yes__ No__ Right__ Left__ Both__

Date: _____

Type: _____

Place of Service: _____

Address: _____

City: _____ State: _____ ZIP: _____

Phone Number: (___) _____

Ultrasound Needed? Yes__ No__ Right__ Left__ Both__

Date: _____
Type: _____
Place of Service: _____
Address: _____
City: _____ State: _____ ZIP: _____
Phone Number: (___) _____
Ultrasound Needed? Yes__ No__ Right__ Left__ Both__

Date: _____
Type: _____
Place of Service: _____
Address: _____
City: _____ State: _____ ZIP: _____
Phone Number: (___) _____
Ultrasound Needed? Yes__ No__ Right__ Left__ Both__

Date: _____
Type: _____
Place of Service: _____
Address: _____
City: _____ State: _____ ZIP: _____
Phone Number: (___) _____
Ultrasound Needed? Yes__ No__ Right__ Left__ Both__

Date: _____
Type: _____
Place of Service: _____
Address: _____
City: _____ State: _____ ZIP: _____
Phone Number: (___) _____
Ultrasound Needed? Yes__ No__ Right__ Left__ Both__

Cervical Screening (Pap Smear)

A cervical screening test is a method of detecting abnormal cells on the cervix. It is done to prevent cervical cancer.

Date: _____
Physician: _____
Place of Service: _____
Address: _____
City: _____ State: _____ ZIP: _____
Phone Number: (___) _____

Date: _____
Physician: _____
Place of Service: _____
Address: _____
City: _____ State: _____ ZIP: _____
Phone Number: (___) _____

Date: _____
Physician: _____
Place of Service: _____
Address: _____
City: _____ State: _____ ZIP: _____
Phone Number: (___) _____

Date: _____
Physician: _____
Place of Service: _____
Address: _____
City: _____ State: _____ ZIP: _____
Phone Number: (___) _____

Cholesterol Test

A cholesterol test checks your blood to see if your cholesterol and triglycerides are at a healthy level.

LDL (low-density lipoprotein)
HDL (high-density lipoprotein)

Date: _____ Total:_____
LDL: _____ HDL: _____ Triglyceride levels: _____

Date: _____ Total:_____
LDL: _____ HDL: _____ Triglyceride levels: _____

Date: _____ Total:_____
LDL: _____ HDL: _____ Triglyceride levels: _____

Date: _____ Total:_____
LDL: _____ HDL: _____ Triglyceride levels: _____

Date: _____ Total:_____
LDL: _____ HDL: _____ Triglyceride levels: _____

Date: _____ Total:_____
LDL: _____ HDL: _____ Triglyceride levels: _____

Date: _____ Total:_____
LDL: _____ HDL: _____ Triglyceride levels: _____

Date: _____ Total:_____
LDL: _____ HDL: _____ Triglyceride levels: _____

Date: _____ Total:_____
LDL: _____ HDL: _____ Triglyceride levels: _____

Colonoscopy

Colonoscopy can detect polyps and early cancers in the intestines.

Date: _____
Place of Service: _____
Address: _____
City: _____ State: _____ ZIP: _____
Phone Number: (___) _____
Ordered by: _____
Result: _____

Date: _____
Place of Service: _____
Address: _____
City: _____ State: _____ ZIP: _____
Phone Number: (___) _____
Ordered by: _____
Result: _____

Date: _____
Place of Service: _____
Address: _____
City: _____ State: _____ ZIP: _____
Phone Number: (___) _____
Ordered by: _____
Result: _____

Diabetes Screening

Diabetes screening is to check for diabetes.

Date: _____   Results: _____
Additional Notes: _____
_____

Date: _____   Results: _____
Additional Notes: _____
_____

Date: _____   Results: _____
Additional Notes: _____
_____

Date: _____   Results: _____
Additional Notes: _____
_____

Date: _____   Results: _____
Additional Notes: _____
_____

Date: _____   Results: _____
Additional Notes: _____
_____

Date: _____   Results: _____
Additional Notes: _____
_____

Other Screenings and/or Tests

Date: _____
Screening/Test: _____
Place of Service: _____
Ordered By: _____
Results: _____
Comments: _____

Date: _____
Screening/Test: _____
Place of Service: _____
Ordered By: _____
Results: _____
Comments: _____

Date: _____
Screening/Test: _____
Place of Service: _____
Ordered By: _____
Results: _____
Comments: _____

Date: _____
Screening/Test: _____
Place of Service: _____
Ordered By: _____
Results: _____
Comments: _____

Date: _____
Screening/Test: _____
Place of Service: _____
Ordered By: _____
Results: _____
Comments: _____

Date: _____
Screening/Test: _____
Place of Service: _____
Ordered By: _____
Results: _____
Comments: _____

Date: _____
Screening/Test: _____
Place of Service: _____
Ordered By: _____
Results: _____
Comments: _____

Date: _____
Screening/Test: _____
Place of Service: _____
Ordered By: _____
Results: _____
Comments: _____

Date: _____
Screening/Test: _____
Place of Service: _____
Ordered By: _____
Results: _____
Comments: _____

Date: _____
Screening/Test: _____
Place of Service: _____
Ordered By: _____
Results: _____
Comments: _____

Date: _____
Screening/Test: _____
Place of Service: _____
Ordered By: _____
Results: _____
Comments: _____

Date: _____
Screening/Test: _____
Place of Service: _____
Ordered By: _____
Results: _____
Comments: _____

Date: _____
Screening/Test: _____
Place of Service: _____
Ordered By: _____
Results: _____
Comments: _____

Date: _____
Screening/Test: _____
Place of Service: _____
Ordered By: _____
Results: _____
Comments: _____

Date: _____
Screening/Test: _____
Place of Service: _____
Ordered By: _____
Results: _____
Comments: _____

Date: _____
Screening/Test: _____
Place of Service: _____
Ordered By: _____
Results: _____
Comments: _____

Date: _____
Screening/Test: _____
Place of Service: _____
Ordered By: _____
Results: _____
Comments: _____

Date: _____
Screening/Test: _____
Place of Service: _____
Ordered By: _____
Results: _____
Comments: _____

Date: _____
Screening/Test: _____
Place of Service: _____
Ordered By: _____
Results: _____
Comments: _____

Date: _____
Screening/Test: _____
Place of Service: _____
Ordered By: _____
Results: _____
Comments: _____

Ask Questions!

It is very important to know the results of your tests. This is *your* health—your body, your *life*.

If you do not understand something, do not be afraid to ask the doctor to explain it. I cannot tell you how many times I have told physicians to talk to me as if I were in the first grade. We have to remember that *they* are in their elements. Medical terminology is their language. This is what they have studied and have been speaking for years, not so for us laypeople.

We have to ask questions, also. If you don't ask questions, the doctors may assume that you know or understand what they are talking about.

On one of my visits, I asked my physician to draw a picture to help me understand what she was telling me. Doctors will usually answer your questions, draw pictures, or print out additional information, if you need it.

Always remember, no question is a dumb question—especially when it involves your health, or that of your loved one.

So, ask away!

Notes

I hope you found *Her Personal Medical Journal* helpful. I am not a doctor, nor do I claim to have any medical education. *Her Personal Medical Journal* is intended to help you keep track of appointments, medications, physicians, and other important information involving your health. It is not meant to replace any files or medical records your physicians or hospitals may have.

You must remember that your physicians only know what you tell them about you. This is especially pertinent if you are rushed to an emergency room, or seeing a particular physician for the first time. The health care provider may ask all types of questions about your health, your history, your medications, the pain, previous procedures, results, etc. The more accurate you are in your answers, the more likely your health care provider will be to accurately diagnose and treat your condition.

I know that every time I go to my primary physician, she reviews my medications. You may have more than one physician, so it is important to keep each of them informed of all the medications you've been prescribed and conditions you have been diagnosed with. You cannot assume that they already know, because they may not.

Remember to take *Her Personal Medical Journal* with you every time you go to see a health care provider. It will also help if you have a trusted person who knows where you keep your *Personal Medical Journal* in case of emergency.

Be Blessed!

www.ingramcontent.com/pod-product-compliance
Lightning Source LLC
Chambersburg PA
CBHW020539290526
45786CB00002B/954